Janet Carr and Roberta Shepherd

EARLY CARE OF THE STROKE PATIENT:

A POSITIVE APPROACH

THIS HANDBOOK HAS BEEN PRODUCED AS A GUIDE TO THE CARE OF PEOPLE IMMEDIATELY FOLLOWING THEIR STROKES, AND IS THEREFORE INTENDED FOR NURSES, RELATIVES, THERAPISTS AND DOCTORS.

William Heinemann Medical Books Ltd

London

First UK edition 1979

being a revised reprint
of the edition first published
in Australia in 1976 entitled
A Positive Approach:
A Handbook for the Early Care
of the Stroke Patient

© Janet Carr and Roberta Shepherd, 1976

ISBN 0 433 30140 6

Reproduced, printed and bound in Great Britain by
Fakenham Press Limited, Fakenham, Norfolk

CONTENTS

ACKNOWLEDGEMENTS

We would like to thank the following people for their invaluable help – Mrs Mary Stephens, Miss Susan Chancellor, Mr Dean Gelding, Mr David Robinson, Mr Ray Howard and Miss Doreen Moore. The photographs on the cover are reproduced with the permission of Miss Josephine Key.

In writing this Handbook, our principle objective is to make practical suggestions as to how to provide an atmosphere in which the hemiplegic patient, immediately following his stroke, will be able to learn to move again as effectively as possible, and so be rehabilitated back into the community.

To do this, all who care for him, relative, nurse, doctor, therapist and social worker, must understand his emotional and physical problems, and the value of motivation. They must understand that physical treatment should commence immediately vital signs are appropriate. They must have some understanding of movement, its dependence on sensation and normal sensory feedback, and of the process by which we learn or relearn a motor skill.

Exercises to the limbs which are passive and to which he does not respond have no place in the early care of this patient. This is not a person with a musculo-skeletal disability who requires improved range at joints or increased strength of muscles. He is a person who requires to learn again how to move. The way to help him to relearn movement is to feed into his brain the sensation of movement and to encourage him to think about the movement he is doing. In this way his brain is stimulated to make the appropriate motor response (figure 1). In other words, it is his brain to which stimulation is directed, not his muscles or limbs.

The four most important factors to understand are:–

1.   The way in which motor skills are learned – basically by repetition, by practice, and by concentration.

2.   The manner in which we perform everyday movements.

3.   The importance of sensory feedback.

4.   The relationship between motivation and learning.

Perhaps we can understand best how motor skills (such as standing up, rolling over in bed, walking) are learned by considering how these movements are first learned by the child. One of the most important factors in the learning of motor skills is the way in which the child prepares himself, very directly and with great attention to detail, for the acquisition of each new skill. For example, he prepares himself for walking very specifically. He begins to develop balance in standing by transferring his weight from one foot to the other in a sideways direction. He cruises sideways around the furniture, and he does this for some time before he has developed sufficient ability to balance on one foot in order to take a step forwards with the other.

Our everyday movements have become so automatic to us over the years of our development and growth that we understand little about them and find it difficult to describe the movements in accurate detail. Doing this requires specially trained skills of observation, plus the use of judgement to evaluate the most essential elements in a particular movement.

For example, the movement from sitting on a stool to standing up involves a particular sequence of events. The feet are brought back under the stool, the head is thrust forwards with the trunk moving forwards from the hips. When the weight is over the feet, the legs and trunk can be extended into the standing position. Throughout the movement weight is symmetrically on both feet and this makes us stable and safe.

Accurate sensory feedback is important in the performance of any movement. We can only move effectively from one position to another if we know where we are in space, and we receive this information from all our sense organs, but particularly from the sense organs in our joints, muscles, skin and balance mechanism of the ear (figure 1).

Physiotherapists helping stroke patients to relearn a certain movement break this movement down into its most important elements and so the patient relearns the movement in the way all motor skills are learned, by practising repeatedly the various elements, and by gradually joining them together into the complete movement. For example, the patient will not be able to take a step forward in standing until he has learned to transfer his weight on to his affected foot and to balance briefly on that foot while he moves the other leg forward. Similarly he will not be able to stand up from his chair effectively until he has practised transferring his weight forwards at his hips.

He will perform the movements more easily and more accurately if he receives accurate sensory information, as this will enable him to monitor his performance. The movement must be explained to him simply and concisely. He should be guided in such a way that he performs the movement correctly. As he improves so he requires less of this manual guidance. He should receive verbal information about the accuracy of the movement — ''Yes, that is correct'' or ''No, let's try again''. It is important that he does not practise movements incorrectly as these will become the movements learned. This of course requires that the patient use all his senses (sight, hearing, touch, position in space) in order that the information his brain receives is as accurate and descriptive as possible.

It is essential that all initial contacts with the patient are positive and effective, leaving him with feelings of hope and anticipation of improvement. He should never be allowed to feel rejected. He should be helped to maintain his sense of importance and of place in his family and in the community. It is at this stage where an intelligent assessment of each individual's problems will ''make a difference between experiencing the patient as a confused old man or seeing him as a human being attempting to come to terms with an overwhelmingly stressful situation'' (Ullman 1964).

His relatives will need help and explanation so they will understand his problems and be able to cope with them. The relatives of a patient with expressive aphasia, for example, will need to understand this problem, so they will not associate it wrongly with intellectual deterioration, and so they will know he is capable of listening and may be able to understand what is said to him.

The approach outlined in this Handbook will enable the hemiplegic patient to co-operate as fully as he can in his rehabilitation, as he will understand what is wrong and what he needs to do about it. He will receive continual help until he can perform the movement himself unaided. He receives encouragement from seeing his small successes because he will understand that these small successes are preparing him for more normal movement and therefore for increasing independence.

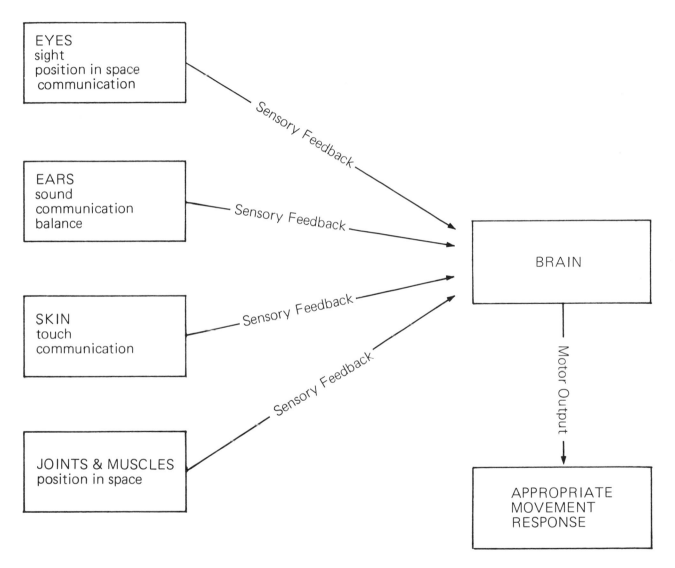

FIGURE 1: THE IMPORTANCE OF SENSATION TO MOVEMENT

OBJECTIVES OF EARLY CARE

To develop an atmosphere in which the patient will be motivated to learn to move again and which will enable him to be rehabilitated within the community.

To reassure relatives and help them understand their important role in the patient's recovery.

To be aware of the patient's frustrations, fears and despair; to give positive help; to be ready to adapt to changes in his emotional state.

To discuss current goals with the patient, his relatives and relevant members of the health professions, so the stimulation of movement (i.e. function) becomes the responsibility of everyone.

To assess and reassess the patient's problems and the approach to these problems so that care will be relevant to each particular patient at the various stages of his progress.

To communicate with the patient and to re-establish as soon as possible more normal oro-facial function.

To discourage compensation with the unaffected side in order to allow the patient to develop movement as symmetrically as possible.

To enable the patient to redevelop his ability to cope with anti-gravity positions as soon as possible. This will help him to reorientate himself with his surroundings, will rewaken the desire to move, and provide the first step towards independence.

To ensure that the patient is given as much opportunity as possible to receive stimulation from his environment.

To prepare the patient for more normal function by concentrating on:

eye-hand contact
weight transference forwards and laterally
weightbearing through the affected arm and leg
symmetrical movement

To give the patient the sensations of normal movements to enable him to relearn these movements.

The methods of teaching movement and restoring function on pages 13 to 53 have been designed to achieve these objectives.

PROBLEMS AND SOME METHODS OF OVERCOMING THEM

The type of problems which may be suffered by a person immediately following a stroke are outlined briefly below.

EMOTIONAL PROBLEMS AND SOCIAL DEPRIVATION

Hopelessness and depression. "The presence of depression coupled with commonly occurring speech disorders and emotional lability may simulate intellectual deterioration even when it does not exist." (Policoff 1970.)

Emotional lability. This is very disturbing for everyone. The patient should be helped to know that his episodes of tearfulness are understood, and are temporary, that as he will regain control over his movements, so also will he gain control over his emotions.

Frustration

Concern about the future

Confusion

This is greatly influenced by the

ATTITUDE OF HOSPITAL STAFF AND RELATIVES

who should strive to demonstrate:

Understanding of the patient's problems.

Awareness of the positive help they can give to enable him to reach his true potential in terms of recovery. This help is given in conjunction with the therapist.

Ability to maintain communication with him despite his speech difficulties. Communication exists in facial expression, hand contact, eye contact, tone of voice, as well as in speech and writing. A positive effort is sometimes required by the inexperienced in order to remember that the patient is neither deaf nor stupid. Communication is essential for the development of a good relationship with the patient.

INCONTINENCE OF BLADDER AND BOWEL

These are frequently present in the early stages, but usually disappear:

1. when the patient stands up, if he is assisted to do this very soon after his stroke, or
2. when he has some means of communicating his need for pan or bottle if he has a speech difficulty.

These two methods will ensure in many cases that catheterisation is unnecessary.

INADEQUATE VENTILATION OF LUNGS

This is only a problem during the short period the patient is confined to bed, i.e. until his vital signs (blood pressure, etc.) are appropriate for increasing activity. It arises to a large extent from the lack of stimulus to take deep breaths. Encouragement and assistance to move around the bed, instead of being passively lifted, will improve ventilation. The physiotherapist will encourage deep breathing by using special techniques.

DISORDERS OF SENSATION

Normal sensation is important for normal movement. The therapist will assess sensation thoroughly and pass on the resultant information to all those caring for the patient. Sensation may be disordered in one or all of the following ways.

There may be failure of sensory impulses from various sense organs (skin, joints, muscles, ears, eyes) to reach the relevant part of the brain, e.g. there may be an inability to recognise where a limb is in space.

There may be difficulty in organising sensation for use in performing movements, e.g. an inability to roll over on the bed when asked, because the patient cannot interpret the various sensations and therefore cannot make the appropriate movement. He may make another movement because he knows he has been asked to do something, but it will be inappropriate. He may be completely unaware of the existence of his affected side, or he may be unaware of his inability to move with his affected side. This may result in his being unable to understand why he is in hospital and why he is having treatment.

Misleading sensory feedback may give him an inappropriate stimulus to move, e.g. if he is allowed to use a lot of effort to perform a movement, in other words to struggle with the movement, he will gradually learn to associate effort with movement. This will prevent him from relearning to move more effectively.

ORO-FACIAL DYSFUNCTION

Disorders of communication may involve any of the following:—

Expressive aphasia, where the patient understands what is said to him but cannot find the right words to speak.

Comprehensive aphasia, where the patient cannot understand what is said to him.

Dysarthria, which is inco-ordination of the muscles used in speaking. This leads to incorrectly spoken words.

Disorders of facial expression may include:—

Asymmetry
Poor lip closure causing dribbling

Disorders of feeding may arise due to:—

Poor lip and jaw closure
Immobile flaccid tongue which is too far forward in the mouth
Poor swallowing
Flaccid cheek allowing food to gather between cheek and gum
Lack of teeth
Difficulty keeping false teeth in position
Poor co-ordination between eating and respiration
Poor head position for eating and drinking. It is impossible to swallow accurately, for example, with the head back

Some of these disorders, if uncorrected, will lead to aspiration and consequent respiratory complications. The therapist will describe the patient's particular problems and give advice about methods of overcoming them (see page 51).

ABNORMAL TONE

Tone is a word used to describe the state of tension as demonstrated in normal muscles. By handling a normal limb, it is possible to develop an understanding of the "feeling" of normal tone.

Most patients have decreased tone on the affected side for a variable period following the stroke. This situation usually changes gradually, and tone becomes either relatively normal or increased beyond the normal. Effective physiotherapy started immediately after the stroke will usually prevent a markedly abnormal increase in tone. In patients whose tone is too high, certain factors, such as anxiety, cold, effort (both mental and physical) will cause an abnormal increase in tone. Decreased tone prevents effective movement as the muscles controlled by the damaged part of the brain are too "limp" to perform the action required. The limbs will feel heavy and unstable. Increased tone results in many movements having to be performed against the resistance of this muscle tone. The factors above (cold, anxiety, effort) will therefore increase the movement difficulty by increasing the tone and therefore the resistance encountered.

PROBLEMS OF MOVEMENT

Poor weight transference
Inability to perform effortless, smooth movement
Difficulty coping with gravity
Inability to bear weight through the limb
Abnormal body alignment

Due to some or all of these factors:

Abnormal tone
Abnormal or absent sensation
Loss of desire to move
Loss of memory of movement
Absence of stimulus to move
Asymmetry
Loss of automatic background to movement, i.e. balance

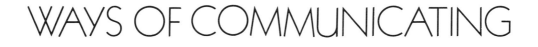

WAYS OF COMMUNICATING

1. Do not discuss the patient or have other conversations in his presence, unless he is also taking part in the discussion.

2. Always look at him and encourage him to look at you. In other words, obtain eye to eye contact.

3. Have relatives present whenever possible. They may be able to communicate with him better than a stranger.

4. Establish whether he speaks English or not, but remember that people sometimes revert to their mother tongue following a stroke.

5. Try to establish a yes/no response and assess whether his inappropriate response is due to diminished or delayed comprehension or inability to select the appropriate response.

6. Give him time to respond or make a sign of response

7. Try to discourage perseveration on one word or phrase.

METHODS OF TEACHING MOVEMENT AND RESTORING FUNCTION

The following photographs are intended to demonstrate methods of improving certain important movements. Where needed, further advice on the individual problems of a particular patient will be given by the therapists involved in the care of that patient.

The subject of these photographs had a hypotonic right hemiplegia at the time this Handbook was produced.

FIGURES 2(a) & 2(b)

Note:

- asymmetrical position of trunk and head
- head facing away from affected side
- affected arm neglected
- difficulty seeing surroundings
- affected shoulder is retracted encouraging the development of increased tone around the shoulder girdle
- patient is too horizontal

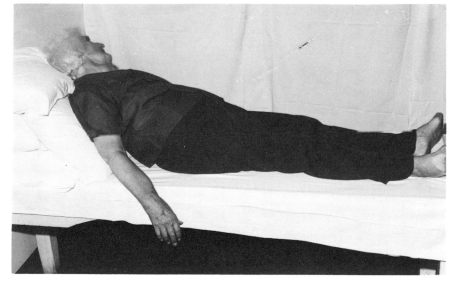

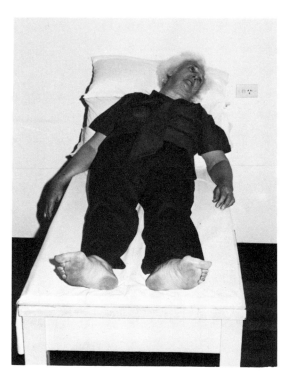

BUT THIS

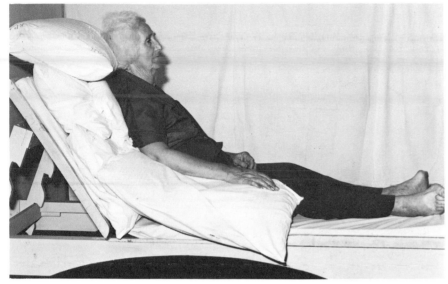

FIGURES 3(a) & 3(b)

Note:

- symmetry of trunk and head
- affected side is easily visible and less likely to be neglected
- affected arm is supported in elevation on a pillow
- affected shoulder is held forwards by small pillow behind the shoulder
- better support allows patient to view her surroundings
- easier position for communication
- hips are more flexed allowing a more upright position

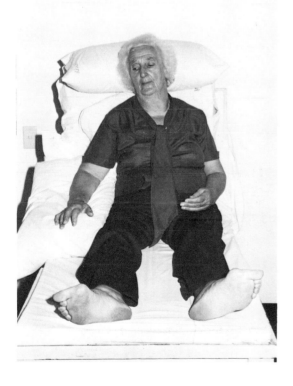

Note:

No monkey grip or overhead ring. Patient is encouraged to move herself about by pushing down on her hands and feet (see figures 5 to 7) which is more natural than pulling up asymmetrically with one hand.

Bed cradle should be used whenever the patient is in bed. It gives her freedom to move about.

Locker on affected side. This allows the patient to reach her belongings by rotating her body to use her unaffected hand. It also keeps her aware of the existence of her affected side.

Patient should be out of bed and sitting in a chair as soon as vital signs allow.

Bed of suitable height. Ideally bed should be of a suitable height to allow patient when sitting on side of bed to have her feet flat on the floor.

Dressing. Patient should be helped to dress as soon as she can sit out of bed. This will improve her morale and gives her a feeling of progress.

ALTERNATIVE POSITIONING IN BED

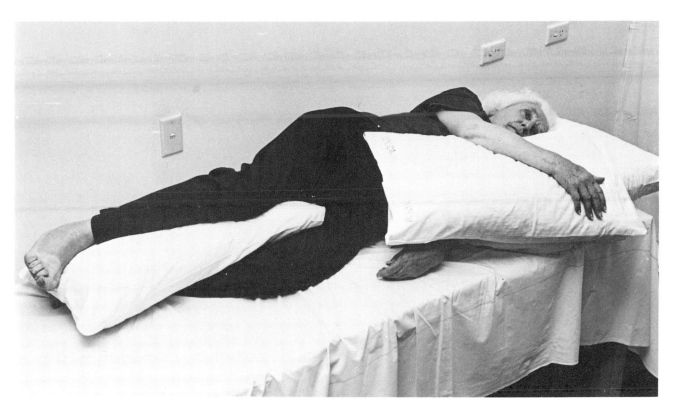

FIGURE 4

Lying on the left side with the affected arm and leg supported forwards on pillows. Positioning like this (as well as in figures 3a and 3b) appears to minimise the development of increased tone which pulls the shoulder back into a retracted position, the arm into flexion and the leg into adduction and internal rotation.

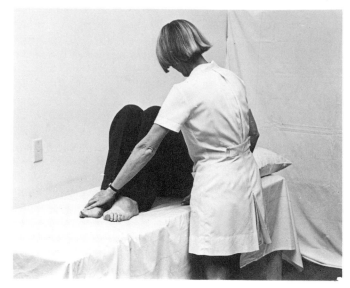

FIGURE 5
Bend both legs at the hips and knees. Hold affected foot flat on the bed.

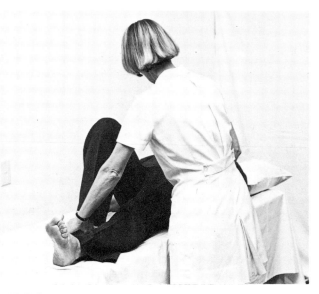

FIGURE 8
With the affected leg bent, roll the pelvis towards you at the same time moving the affected shoulder forwards. Patient should then be lying on her side.

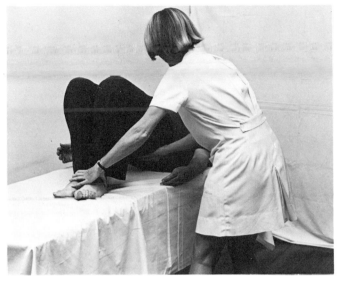

FIGURE 6
Ask patient to lift her bottom up and to the right side, then down. She should try to push down on both feet and arms.

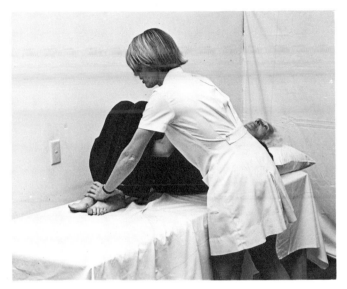

FIGURE 7
Move her shoulders and feet across. Patient should try to do some of the movement herself but not with undue effort.

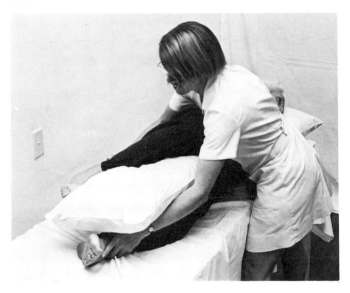

FIGURE 9
Support the affected leg on a pillow in a slightly flexed position, and the affected arm on another pillow with the shoulder forwards and arm extended as in figure 4.

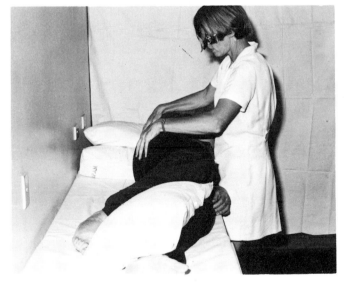

FIGURE 10
In this position the patient should try to roll her hip forwards in order to get the feeling of controlling her position.

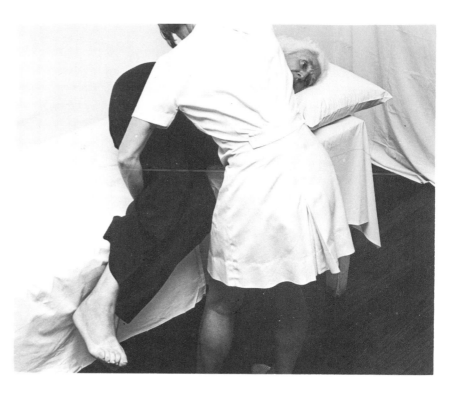

FIGURE 11
Swing her legs over the side of the bed.

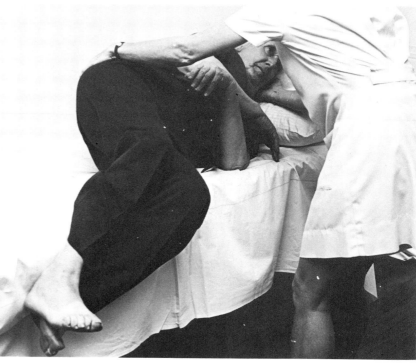

FIGURE 12
Ask the patient to lift her head up sideways and encourage her to feel how she does this movement. At the same time she should also try to push down with her right hand.

SITTING ON SIDE OF BED

Assist the patient to the side of the bed as in figures 5 to 7. She should be nearer the side of the bed from which she is getting out. Help her to turn on to her side as in figure 8.

Note: The movement can also be done with the unaffected side uppermost.

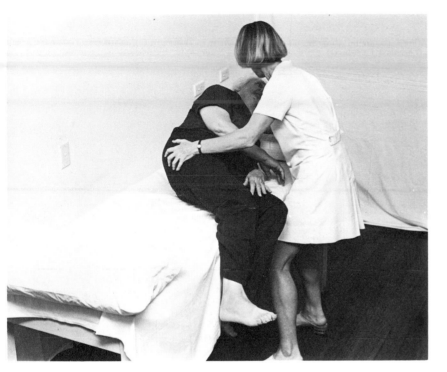

FIGURE 13
With one hand lifting her under the left shoulder and the other pushing down on the right side of the pelvis,

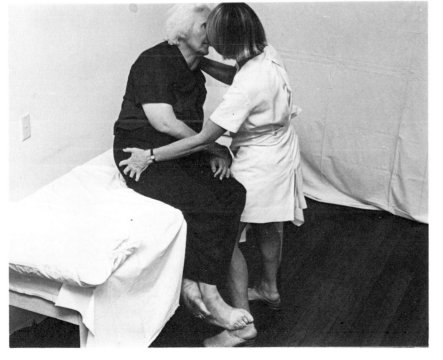

FIGURE 14
help her to sit up by shifting her weight towards the right and by encouraging her to move her head to the right. Remind her to keep her weight forwards at the hips.

21

NOT THIS

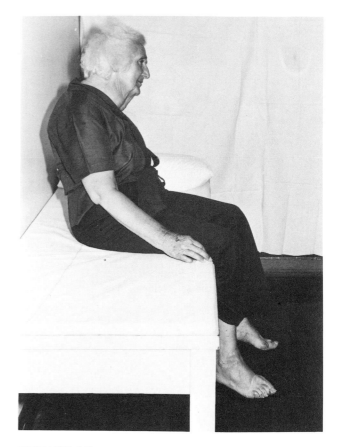

FIGURE 15
Without help this is how the patient sits. Her weight is too far back and over to the unaffected side.

TRANSFERRING WEIGHT IN SITTING

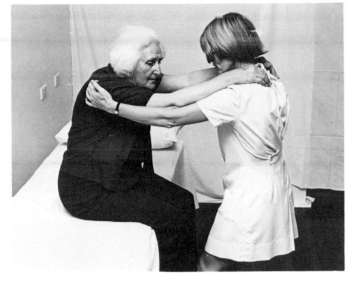

FIGURE 16
Practise weight transference forwards,

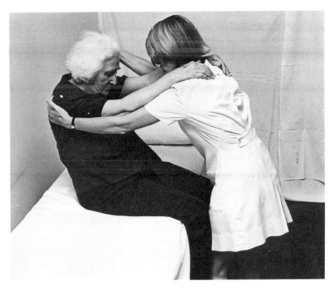

FIGURE 17
and backwards at the hips, with righting of the head.*

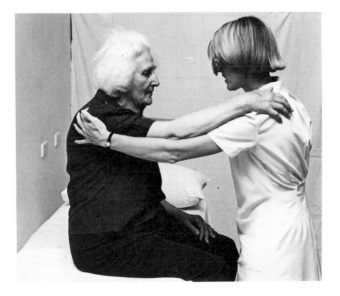

FIGURE 18
Patient now tries to sit with her weight forwards.

*Head righting.
Normally when transferring weight forwards in sitting the head extends, and when transferring weight backwards it flexes.

NOT THIS

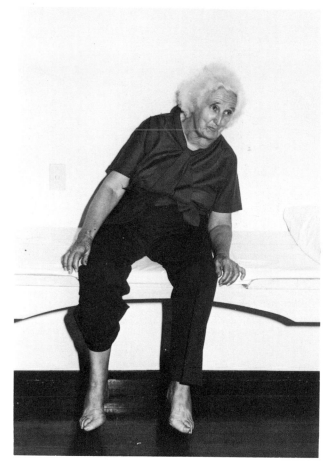

FIGURE 19
Without help the patient may tend to fall to one side.

TRANSFERRING WEIGHT IN SITTING

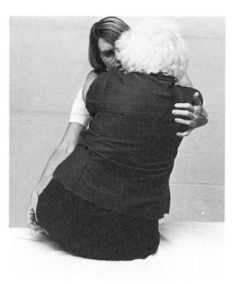

FIGURE 20
Practise weight transference to the right side. Right shoulder is kept elevated. Stimulation to the left side of her bottom will encourage hitching of the hip.

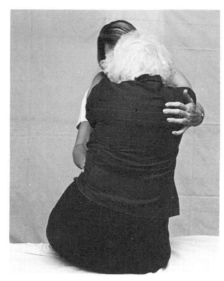

FIGURE 21
Gentle pressure at the waist will also encourage hip hitching.

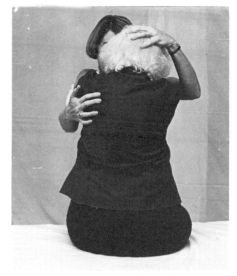

FIGURE 22
Practise weight transference to the left side. If the patient does not right her head laterally* she should be helped to do so.

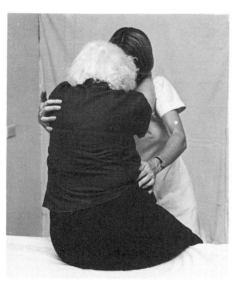

FIGURE 23
Gentle pressure at the waist will encourage hip hitching.

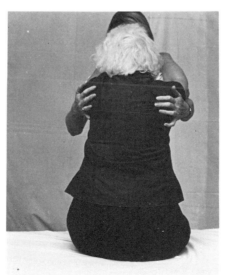

FIGURE 24
The patient gets the feeling of a symmetrical position. Her weight is kept well forwards at the hips.

*Head righting.
Normally when transferring weight to one side in sitting, the head moves sideways in the opposite direction.

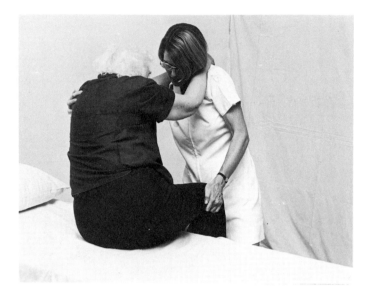

FIGURE 25
Combine transferring weight forwards and to the left with hitching the pelvis up on the right.

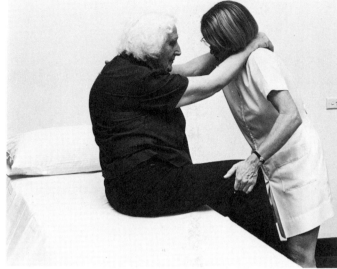

FIGURE 26
Bring the right leg forwards. Repeat from side to side

STANDING UP FROM BED

Practise weight transference forwards and sideways as in figures 16 to 24.

FIGURE 27
until the patient is on the edge of the bed with feet on the floor.

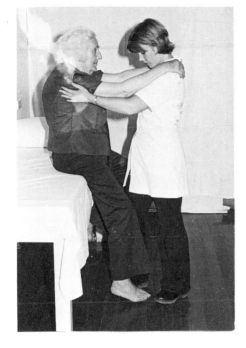

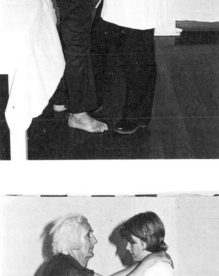

FIGURE 28
Stand her up with some weight on the affected side. Keep the pelvis forwards and encourage her to keep her knee straight. Support her knee with your knee intermittently if necessary.

FIGURE 29
Elevate shoulder to improve symmetry.

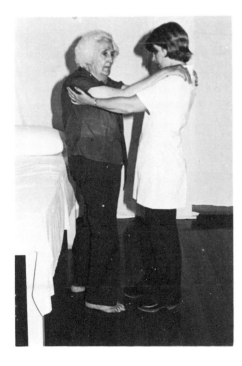

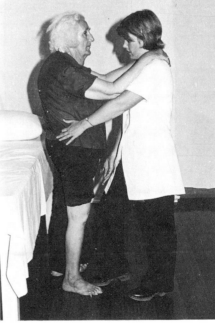

FIGURE 30
Encourage her to keep her pelvis forwards, knee straight and her weight on the affected side.

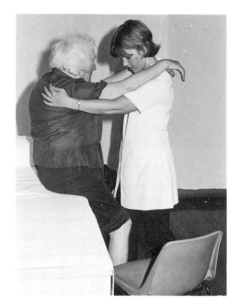

FIGURE 31
Place chair at an angle to the bed on the affected side. Have the patient's arm resting gently on your shoulders in extension. She should not pull down on your shoulders.

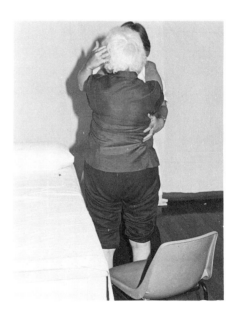

FIGURE 35
Gentle pressure to the waist will encourage hip hitching. Ask her to take a step to the right side. You can help place her foot with your foot if necessary.

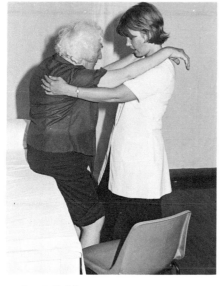

FIGURE 32
Feet on to the floor.

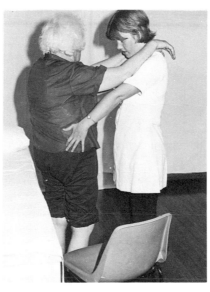

FIGURE 33
Ask patient to stand up bringing her pelvis, and therefore her weight, forwards.

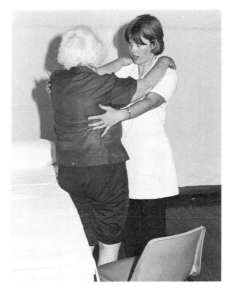

FIGURE 34
Transfer weight on to the left side and hitch the right hip.

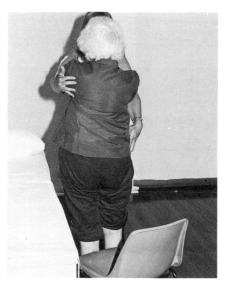

FIGURE 36
Her weight is on the left side. She should transfer some of her weight back on to the right side to gain symmetry.

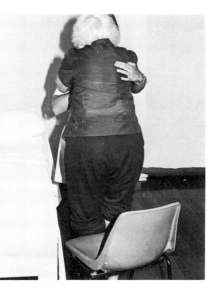

FIGURE 37
Transfer weight backwards by bending forwards at the hips.

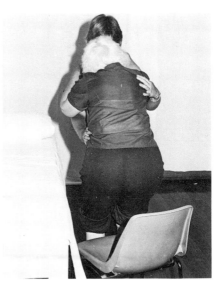

FIGURE 38
Ask her to push her bottom backwards and sit down.

METHOD 1

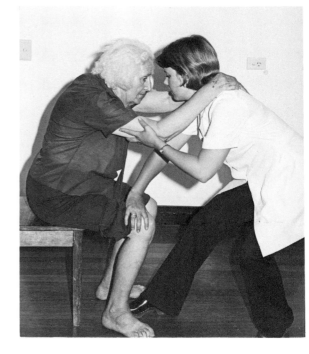

FIGURE 39
Make sure both feet are well back. Transfer weight forwards at the hips. Place your opposite hand on the affected knee and keep the right shoulder elevated.

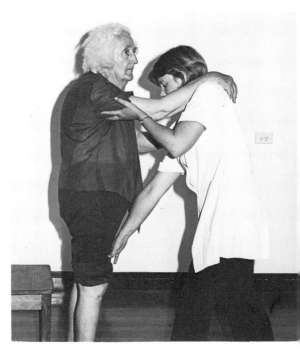

FIGURE 40
Ask the patient to stand up while you help her transfer weight on to the affected leg. Encourage patient to get her pelvis forwards with the knee straight.

STANDING UP FROM CHAIR

METHOD 2

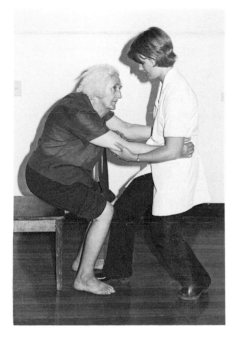

FIGURE 41
Feet well back. Weight forwards at the hips.

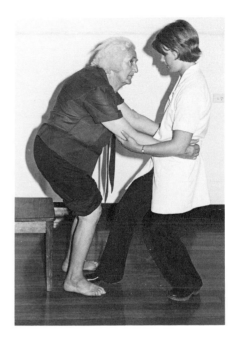

FIGURE 42
Patient to concentrate on lifting her bottom up. This will help her to keep her weight forwards.

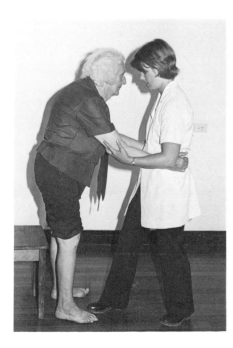

FIGURE 43
Hips, and therefore weight, are too far back and she is unstable.

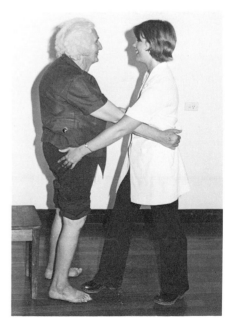

FIGURE 44
Patient is encouraged and helped to move her pelvis forwards. This brings her weight forwards and makes her more stable.

SITTING DOWN ON CHAIR

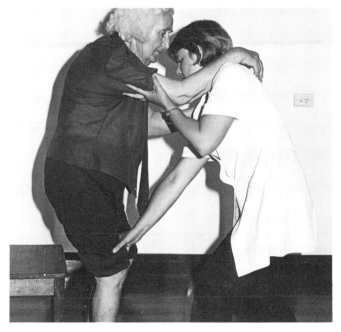

FIGURE 45
Ask the patient to bend at the hips.

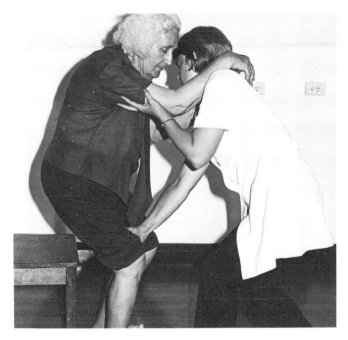

FIGURE 46
Patient should think about pushing her bottom backwards. This will bend the hips sufficiently to enable her to transfer her weight backwards and sit down.

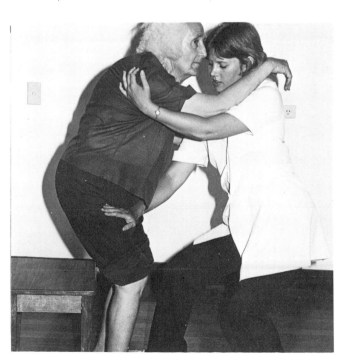

Alternative Method
This is used when the patient has difficulty in bending the hips and transferring her weight backwards.

FIGURE 47
Pressure downwards and backwards on the thigh plus the instruction to push her bottom backwards will help the patient understand the movement required.

NOT THIS

FIGURES 48(a) & 48(b)

Note:

Asymmetrical position of trunk and head

Head facing away from affected side

Affected arm neglected

Insufficient hip flexion therefore weight too far backwards

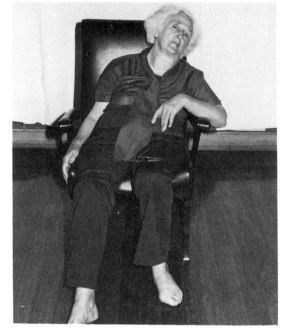

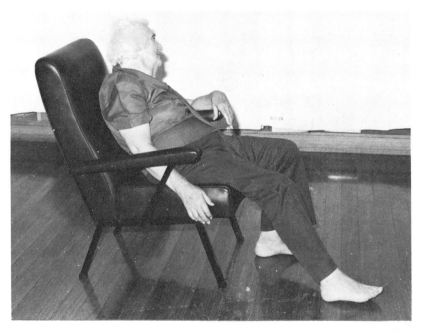

SITTING

Firm chair of a suitable height to enable the patient's feet to rest on the floor.

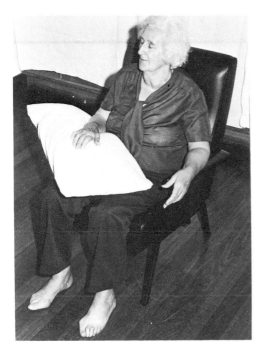

FIGURES 49(a) & 49(b)
Note:
Symmetry of trunk and head.
Hips flexed therefore weight further forwards
Affected shoulder elevated
Both feet flat on floor
Patient is able to look around

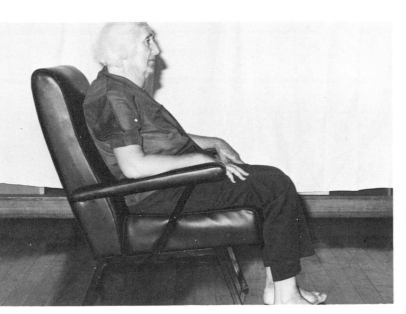

ALTERNATIVE POSITION

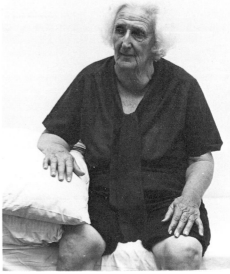

FIGURE 50

Note:
Symmetry of trunk and head
Affected shoulder elevated

NOT THIS

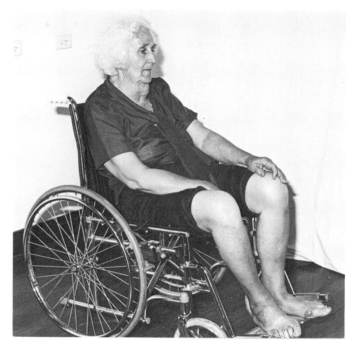

FIGURE 51
Poor positioning in wheelchair.
Note:
Asymmetry of trunk and head
Weight too far backwards

BUT THIS

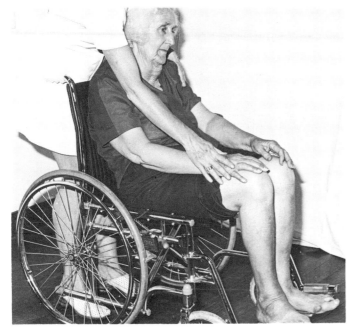

FIGURE 52
Improve symmetry,

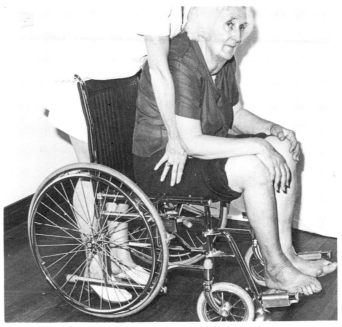

FIGURE 53
then transfer weight forwards by flexing her hips.
Ask patient to move her bottom backwards.

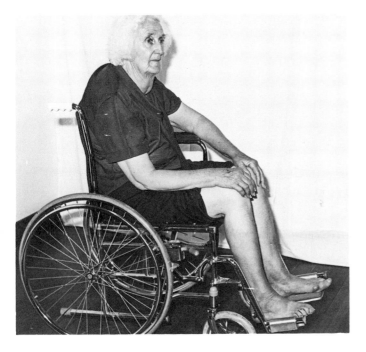

FIGURE 54
Improved sitting position with hips well back in
chair.

In order to take a step forwards it is necessary to transfer the weight sideways on to one leg.

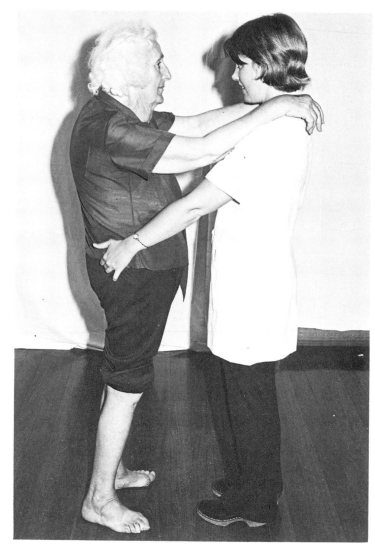

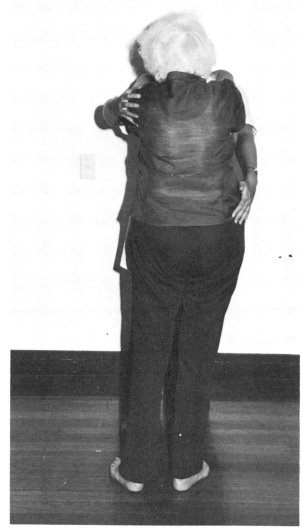

FIGURE 55

This follows on from figures 30 and 44. Patient is standing with pelvis forwards and weight equally distributed on both feet. Her hands resting on the therapist's shoulders give her confidence and support when these are needed.

FIGURE 56

Transferring weight to the right side. Patient must keep shoulders level and transfer her weight by moving the pelvis a small distance to the right. Therapist's left hand is controlling the extent of the movement.

TRANSFERRING WEIGHT SIDEWAYS IN STANDING

IN PREPARATION FOR WALKING

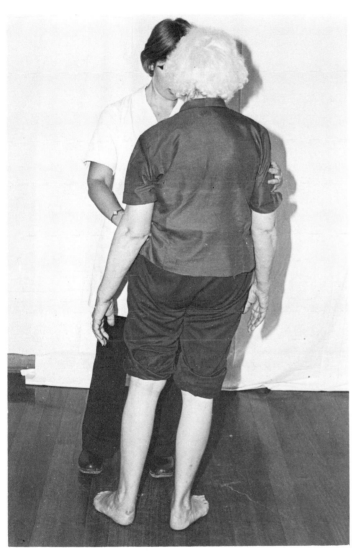

FIGURE 57
The movement of transferring weight can be encouraged by stimulating the side of the trunk above the pelvis.

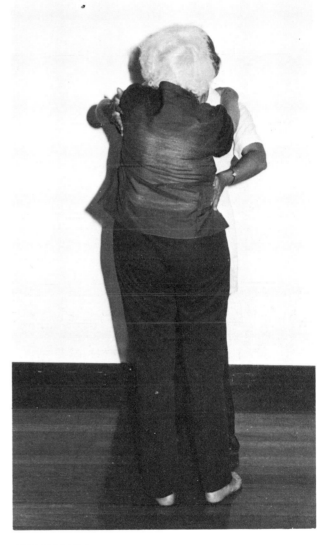

FIGURE 58
Transferring weight to the left side. Therapist's left hand encourages the movement.

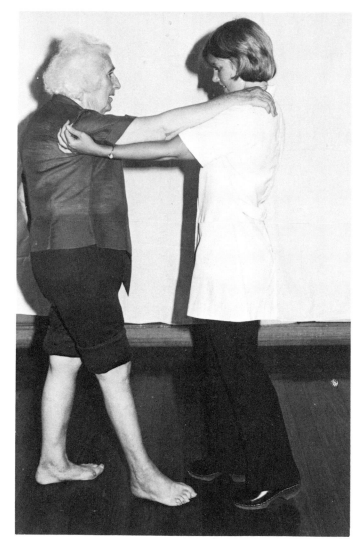

FIGURE 59
Patient is standing with affected leg forwards. Her weight is too far back and is still on the left leg.

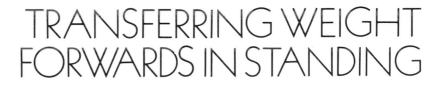

TRANSFERRING WEIGHT FORWARDS IN STANDING

IN PREPARATION FOR WALKING

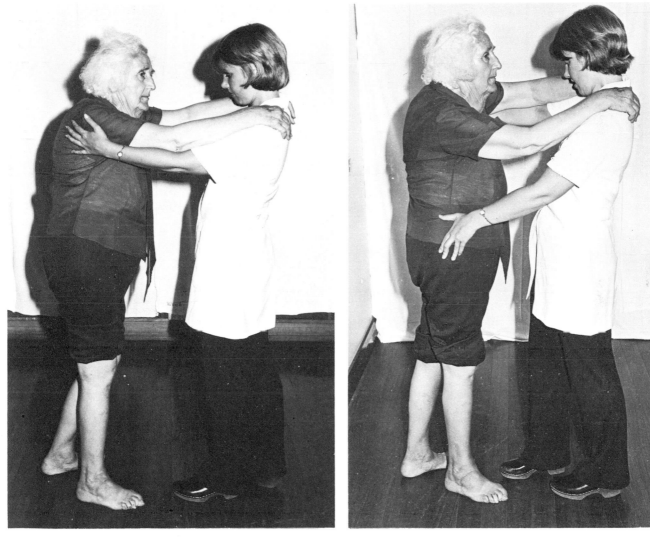

FIGURE 60
She has tried to transfer her weight forwards, but instead has bent forwards at the hips, which leaves her weight too far back. She is also bending her left knee which should remain straight.

FIGURE 61
She is helped to transfer her weight by moving her pelvis forwards until her weight is over the right foot.

Note:
When the patient has understood what is required in figure 61 she is asked to step forwards and backwards with the left leg. This helps her appreciate the feeling of weight-bearing on the right leg.

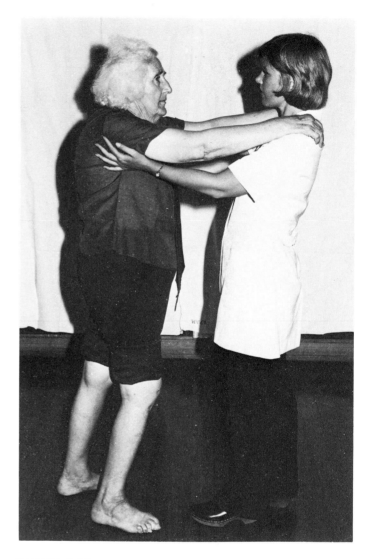

FIGURE 62
She has difficulty transferring weight on to the affected leg because of instability of her right knee.

IN PREPARATION FOR WALKING

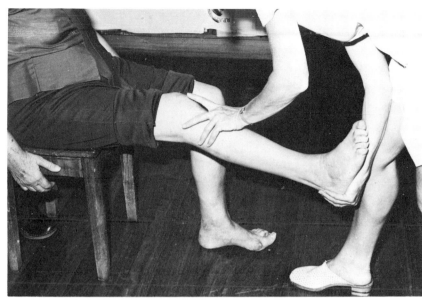

FIGURE 63
Sit the patient on a stool. Extend her leg but do not hold her knee and do not let it hyperextend. Ask the patient to keep her knee straight while you apply strong pressure through the heel in the direction of the hip. Then ask the patient to bend her knee a little and straighten it again. This will help her to control her knee in the small range required for weight-bearing on the leg.

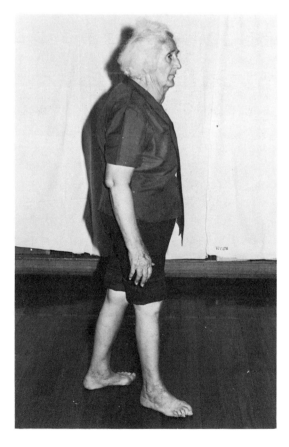

FIGURE 64
Assist her to stand up. She is now able to control her knee.

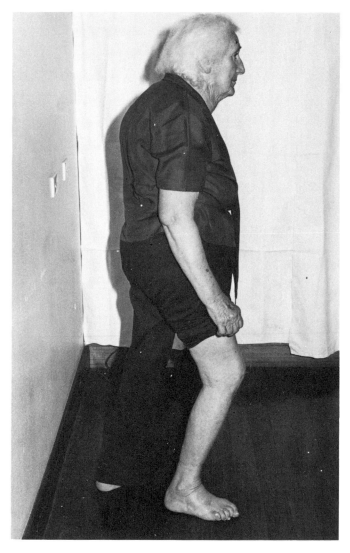

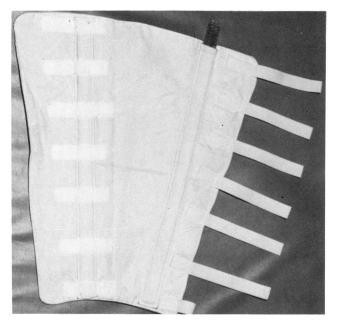

FIGURE 66
A calico splint with two or three metal struts and Velcro straps can be used for a few days to give the patient the feeling of stability and to enable her to practise weight transference.

FIGURE 65
Patient is unable to transfer her weight on to her affected leg because of instability of the knee.

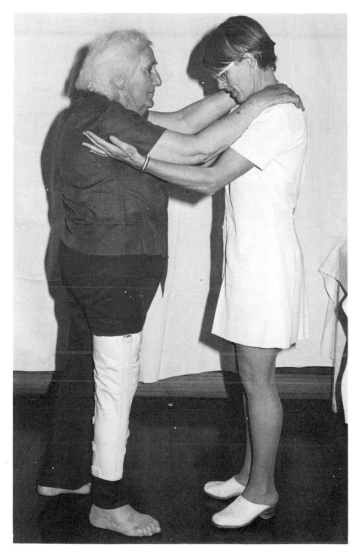

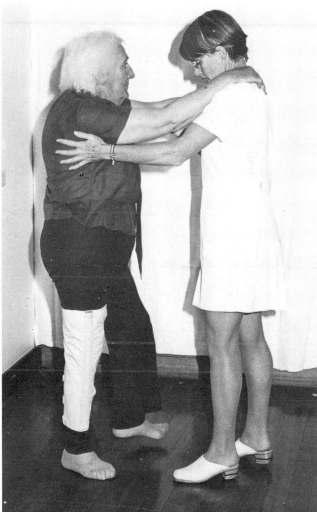

FIGURE 67
Practising weight transference in standing with pelvis well forwards.

FIGURE 68
She is now stable enough to take a step forwards with the unaffected leg.

Note:
After the patient has practised this a few times, take the splint off and see if she can control her knee herself.

METHOD 1

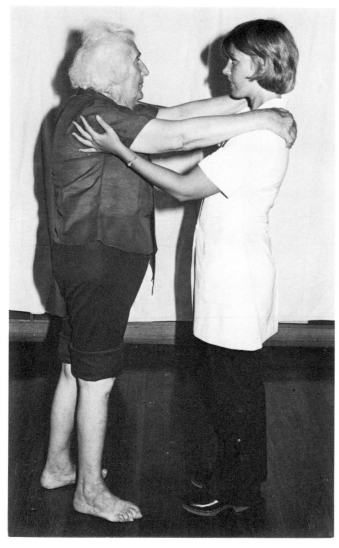

FIGURE 69
This follows on from figure 61. The patient's hands are resting on the therapist's shoulders to give confidence and some stability.

METHOD 2

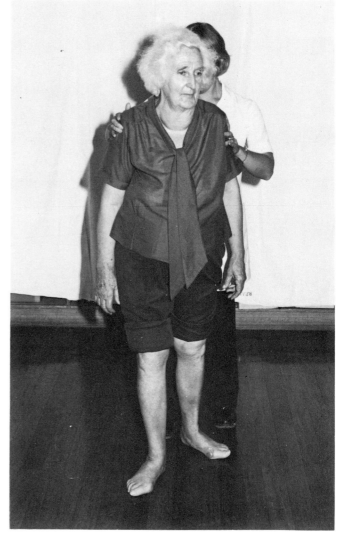

FIGURE 70
Holding the shoulders lightly, transfer her weight gently sideways and forwards on to the right leg, at the same time moving the right shoulder forwards.

METHOD 3

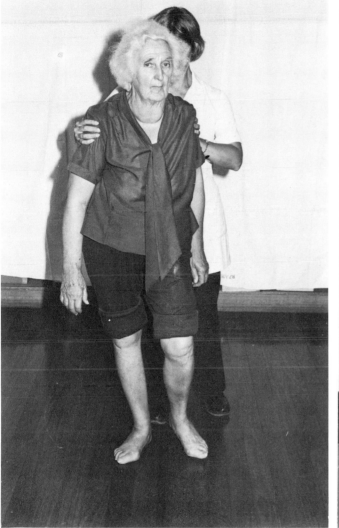

FIGURE 71
She is now able to take a step with her left leg.

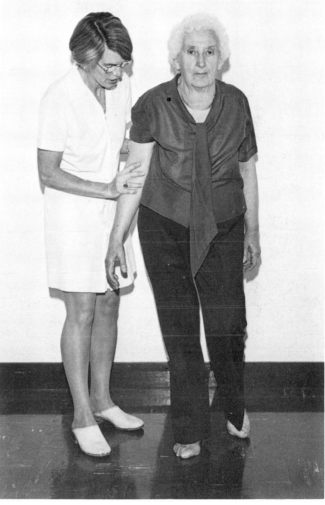

FIGURE 72
Elevation of the affected shoulder may be sufficient help for the patient. Note the therapist's hand on the upper arm.

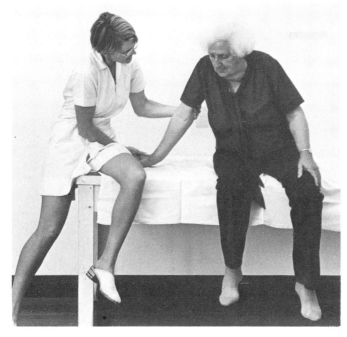

FIGURE 73
Therapist encourages patient to transfer her weight towards the right side, keeping the elbow straight and shoulder elevated. Patient should think about bearing weight through her hand, with her weight on the right side of her bottom.

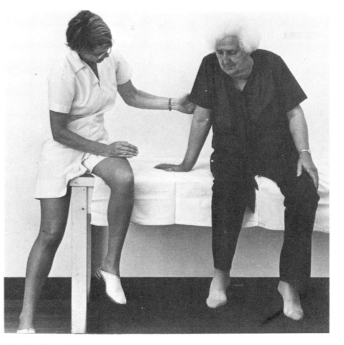

FIGURE 74
She can now keep her weight over on the right side if her elbow is gently supported. Give only the minimal assistance to enable the patient to maintain the position. Make sure she keeps her weight forwards at the hips.

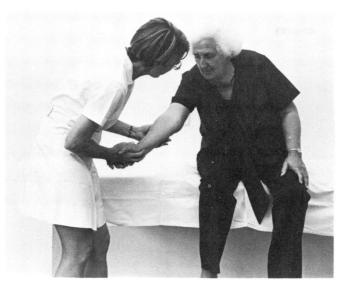

FIGURE 75
Patient can now attempt to transfer her weight forwards as well as laterally. This helps her develop her confidence in moving around.

WEIGHT BEARING THROUGH THE ARM

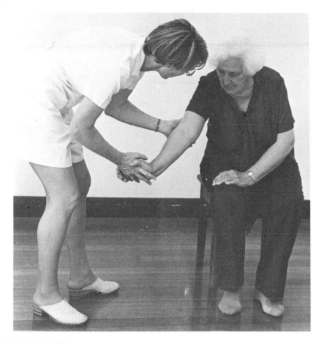

FIGURE 76
A progression from figure 75. Patient can now practise transferring her weight much further forwards and this increases her confidence in sitting.

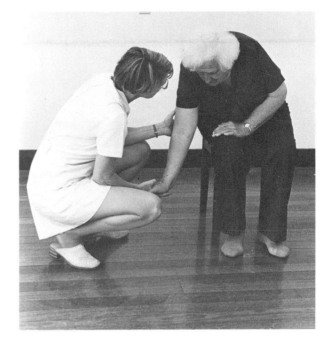

FIGURE 77
Make sure that the shoulder is kept elevated. This will encourage her to transfer her weight forwards.

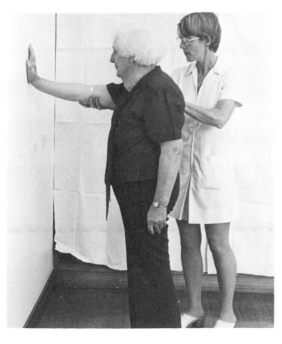

FIGURE 78
It is important that the patient gains some control around the shoulder girdle with the arm in an elevated position. This will prepare her for reaching and grasping. Weight-bearing through the arm in this position helps to stimulate more control.

1. The patient should be in a sitting position (see page 35). It is difficult and dangerous to swallow fluids or solids with the head back or while lying down, because the patient may choke.

2. It is easier to cope with solid food (e.g. food the consistency of firm mashed potato) than fluids, so start with these if he is having difficulty eating.

3. Make sure he has food he likes. To increase his awareness of what is in his mouth, foods of different texture should be given to him.

4. A patient who normally wears false teeth should wear them again as soon as he is able to retain them safely. If they are left out for too long, changes to his mouth result in poor fitting and consequent need for a replacement set.

5. Sit yourself to the affected side of the patient or directly in front of him.

6. Make sure he can breathe through his nose before you encourage lip closure. Remember that nose blowing is usually a bi-manual task.

7. For the following procedures your fingers used gently and firmly are your best tools, as they will give you sensory feedback about what is happening.

METHODS OF OVERCOMING ORO-FACIAL PROBLEMS

PROBLEM

SUGGESTION

1. **Poor or uneven lip closure**
   Facial asymmetry

   (i) Hold jaw closed.
   (ii) Briskly stroke the affected side of the face in direction of lip closure.
   N.B. If the unaffected side of the face is overactive, encourage him to relax this side.

2. **Ineffective swallowing**
   Drooling

   (i) Place your finger on the anterior third of tongue, pushing it down and back. This will elevate the posterior third of tongue sealing the oral cavity.
   (ii) Withdraw finger.
   (iii) Hold jaw lightly closed
   (iv) Ask him to swallow.

3. **Poor chewing**

   (i) Sensation of food in mouth may stimulate chewing.
   (ii) Hold jaw in a lightly closed position and rotate in a chewing movement, and move it from side to side.

4. **Difficulty drinking**
   N.B. Fluids are more easily aspirated than solids, so it is better to give him solid food first as this will help prepare him for fluids.

   (i) Improve lip closure as above.
   (ii) Place cup on lower lip (a plastic cup with lip may be easier) and allow a small amount of fluid to enter the mouth.
   (iii) Stimulate lip closure as above, while reminding him to swallow.

5. **Food trapped persistently between cheek and gum**
   (This is due to poor tone in the buccinator muscle.)

   (i) Briskly stroke affected cheek in an upwards direction to stimulate tone.

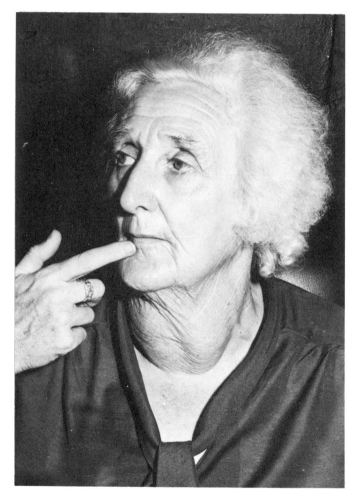

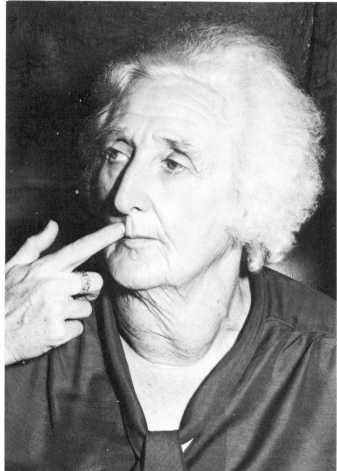

FIGURE 79
Improve lip closure on the affected side by stroking the bottom lip up and towards the midline,

FIGURE 80
and by stroking the top lip down and towards the midline.

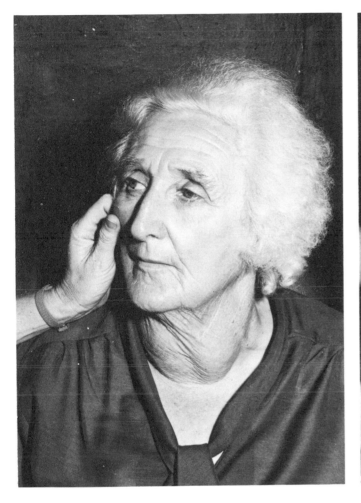

FIGURE 81
Improve tone in the cheek by stroking upwards from the corner of the lip towards the eye.

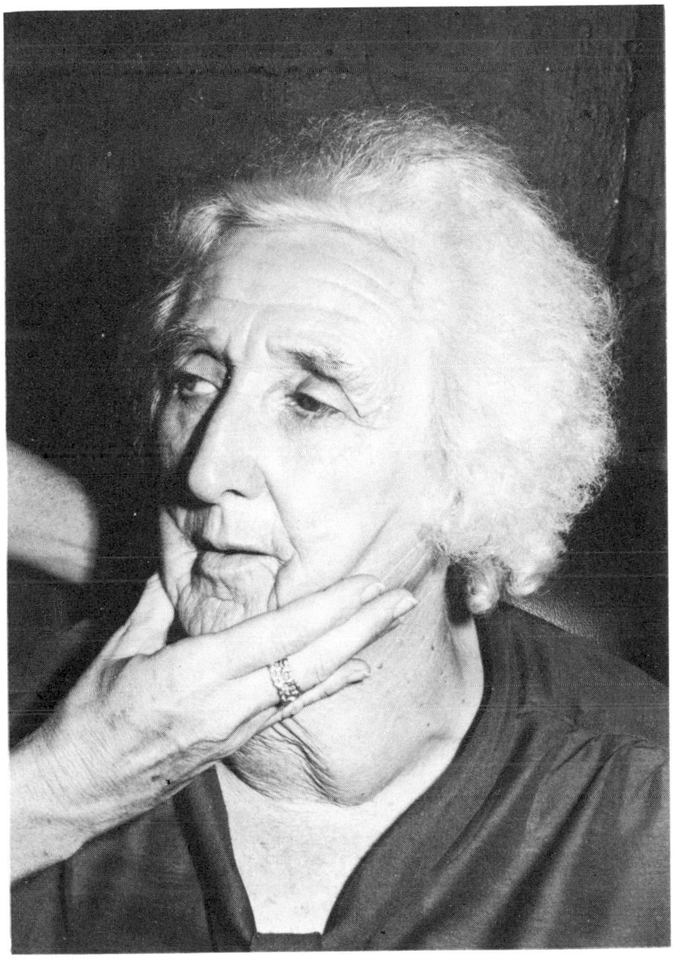

FIGURE 82
Stimulate chewing by placing food in the mouth and gently moving the bottom jaw.

REFERENCES

BOBATH, B. (1978) Adult Hemiplegia 2nd edn. London: Heinemann.

POLICOFF, L. D. (1970) The philosophy of stroke rehabilitation. *Geriatrics* 25, 99.

ULLMAN, M. (1964) Disorders of body image after stroke. *Am. J. of Nursing* 64, 10, 89.